HERBAL MEDICINE FOR SLEEP AND RELAXATION

by Dr Desmond Corrigan

B.Sc (Pharmacy), M.A., Ph.D., F.L.S., F.P.S.I.

Published by
Amberwood Publishing Ltd
Park Corner, Park Horsley, East Horsley, Surrey KT24 5RZ
Tel: 01483 285919

ISBN 1-899308-07-5

Typeset and designed by
Word Perfect, Christchurch, Dorset.

Cover design by Design Hive

Printed in Great Britain

PLANTLIFE

Thr Natural History Museum, Cromwell Road, London SW7 5BD

Registered Charity No. 328576

Amberwood Publishing supports the Plantlife Charity,
Britain's only charity exclusively dedicated to saving wild plants.

CONTENTS

Note to Reader

Whilst the author has made every effort to ensure that the contents of this book are accurate in every particular, it is not intended to be regarded as a substitute for professional medical advice under treatment. The reader is urged to give careful consideration to any difficulties which he or she is experiencing with their own health and to consult their General Practitioner if uncertain as to its cause or nature. Neither the author nor the publisher can accept any legal responsibility for any health problem which results from use of the self-help methods described.

About the Author

Senior Lecturer and Head of the Department of Pharmacognosy, School of Pharmacy, University of Dublin, Trinity College, Ireland.

Dr. Corrigan was born and educated in Dublin. After obtaining his degree in Pharmacy he spent some time in the pharmaceutical industry before joining the staff of the School of Pharmacy. Dr. Corrigan is a former analyst with the Drug Squad of the Irish Police and since 1980 he has been deeply involved in community drug education and other drug prevention activities. He is author of "Facts about Drug Abuse in Ireland", now in its Third Edition. Dr. Corrigan's research is concentrated in the area of phytotherapy, in particular, aspects of the quality control of phytomedicines and the testing of herbal medicines. Dr. Corrigan has lectured at many national and international conferences on phytotherapy. He is co-chairman of the Scientific Committee of ESCOP – the European Scientific Cooperative on Phytotherapy – and a member of the Editorial Advisory Boards of the International Journal of Pharmacognosy, the British Journal of Phytotherapy and the European Journal of Herbal Medicine.

Foreword

'Herbs and plants are medical jewels gracing the woods, fields and lanes which few see, and few minds understand. Through this want of observation and knowledge the world suffers immense loss.'

(Linnaeus, 1707-1778)

Little has changed in the passing years; as Culpepper noted even before, ". . . the great mass of (medical) practitioners at the present day are as ignorant of the science of Botany as the horses on which they ride. No medical man should consider his education complete without a knowledge of Botany." With this monograph on *Herbal Medicine for Sleep and Relaxation*, the author has brought together a wealth of information which would comfort Linnaeus and Culpepper.

Here is a distillation of the history and science of the herbs commonly associated with sleep, that makes interesting reading as well as an interesting resource. As Dr Corrigan points out in his introduction, very many people have taken a prescribed sleeping pill in the previous years; but the problem is even more pervasive. Insomnia is the most common of all sleep disorders. A third of the adult population, both male and female is affected, at least occasionally. Of adult patients experiencing insomnia, only 5% seek professional help, even though 9% to 17% of these patients consider their insomnia serious. Of those seeking help as many as 20% receive no treatment at all, despite the fact that the history of insomnia is a predictor of future insomnia. Sleep loss exhibits potent effects on the individual experiencing sleeplessness and causes decreasing cognitive abilities, alertness and work performance after even a short period of impairment. Fatigue experienced during the day following loss of sleep is dangerous physically, emotionally and economically not only to the affected individual, but to society as a whole. As also pointed out in the introduction, treatment with hypnotic drugs is common, particularly in those over the age of sixty-five, but many more patients self-medicate with alcohol and over-the-counter products such as antihistamines, whilst others continue to suffer.

How is it that nature, which has given us almost all the magic bullets we possess such as antibiotics and anti-cancer drugs, has been all but ignored in sleep. The development of Complementary Medicine, the study and teaching of non-orthodox, non-allopathic remedies such as acupuncture, manipulation and of course herbal compounds, is now a part of the medicine curriculum and may help resolve this issue. In the USA 40% of medical schools have courses in such fields, whilst in the UK, although far fewer medical schools are involved, a newly created Chair of Complementary Medicine in Exeter as well as two new degree courses has made the study of herbal remedies in particular legitimate. Again, from Culpepper, "The study of botany is a delightful one. The exercise in collecting plants invigorates the health, and the intellectual qualities. Botany also is extensively applied to useful purposes. From the vegetable kingdom derives a large share of sustenance, and from the same source he derives agents for the cure of his complaints."

Herbal Medicine for Sleep and Relaxation is a resource for our times. All those with an interest in the simple and safe induction of restful sleep will be amply rewarded with new ideas, and agreeable and effectual remedies.

Adrian J Williams FRCP
October 1995

1 | Introduction

Like many other things in life we take for granted our ability to temporarily hibernate every day. However, deprive us of our customary 'shut eye' and even those resolute souls who can tolerate all sorts of discomfort begin to suffer. We seem to be obsessed with sleep or, more correctly, the lack of it. For example the Oxford Dictionary of Quotations includes 57 quotations about sleep. It is estimated that in the U.K. about one in five adults claim not to get as much sleep as they would like. Insomnia, that feeling of excessive wakefulness at night, is often treated with hypnotic drugs and surveys show that 4% of adults and 16% of those over 65 had taken a "sleeping pill" in the previous year.

Prescribing of what are called the benzodiazepine hypnotics is widespread. These well-known drugs are also used to treat anxiety. The fact that they are remarkably safe in terms of overdosage initially resulted in a complacent attitude to their safety. However there is a price to be paid for the useful effects of drugs such as Diazepam and its many relatives. Dependence or addiction may develop after 4-6 weeks of continuous use. Side effects, such as daytime drowsiness, headache, poor concentration, reduced memory and reaction times, are common. Other hazards include falls and fractures and these drugs can affect our ability to drive or operate machinery, both immediately and through a hangover effect the following day. Thankfully the risks of these drugs are now more widely understood and the advice from the Committee on the Safety of Medicines (CSM) states quite clearly that "Benzodiazepines should be used to treat insomnia only when it is severe, disabling or subjecting the individual to extreme distress". Medical advice states that these drugs should not be given for more than three weeks (preferably for only one week).

Given the justifiable concern over the indiscriminate use of these sleeping pills, what alternatives are there for the many who suffer from mild occasional or even longer-term insomnia? Sensible prevention in the form of avoidance of caffeinated drinks and alcohol before bedtime can help. Massage, aromatherapy, relaxation techniques, even sex, have all been recommended as non-drug alternatives.

Naturally, many people look to plants and herbs for a remedy to their sleeplessness. To some this might seem strange but many herbs can contain the promise of a good night's sleep. It is not for nothing that the latin botanical name for the opium poppy is *Papaver somniferum* — somniferum meaning 'sleep bearing' and that the powerful drug morphine from that poppy is named after Morpheus the God of Sleep. Not that one would recommend using either opium or morphine for insomnia, but there are other plants which could provide a safe effective alternative, not just to the juice of the poppy but also to the synthetic drugs, all too frequently resorted to by those in search of

> "Sleep that knits up the ravell'd sleave of care,
> The death of each day's life, sore labours bath,
> Balm of hurt minds, great natures second course,
> Chief nourisher in lifes feast."
> [From the Scottish play by W. Shakespeare].

In the following chapters we look at these herbs in detail, showing how modern science reinvents the wheel by validating what our forebears knew well, namely, that herbs such as Valerian, Passiflora, Hops and many more, do provide a safe gentle way of helping those of us who find a decent night's sleep elusive.

1 | Valerian – a star among stars

It is difficult to imagine anything which smells worse than the roots of the Valerian plant. Not surprisingly, the ancient Greek and Roman physicians called it *Phu*! Yet this plant, which has been used as a medicine for at least two thousand years, is still, despite its smell, one of the key herbal drugs of the late 20th century. The past few years have seen more than 200 scientific papers on Valerian attempting to describe its properties. It has proven to be not only a popular herb but also a safe and effective herb ever since those classical doctors first used it.

The name Valeriana was first used around the 10th century and it seems to have been the Anglo-Saxon leeches who first showed real appreciation of its virtues. By the 17th century Valerian was well established and the great English herbalist, Nicholas Culpeper, described Valerian under four separate headings. Under the heading Greek Valerian he wrote that "it helps in nervous complaints, head–aches, trembling palpitations of the heart, vapours and all that train of miserable disorders included under the name of nervous."

Scientific medicine has always valued Valerian even when other herbs became less important or even scorned. The plant, known botanically as *Valeriana officinalis*, has always been officially recognised in the Pharmacopoeias, the recognised compendia of quality standards for drugs. Valerian is described in the European and British Pharmacopoeias at the present time. Not surprisingly, pharmaceutical and medical scientists have spent much time investigating this plant and the results show why this plant deserves its superstar status.

By Way of Background

A recent television food programme featured a product whose claim to fame included the fact that it contained 'phytochemicals'. Well of course every plant contains phytochemicals because the word 'phyto' is derived from the Greek word for plant, so phytochemical simply means a plant chemical. Some of these plant chemicals are essential to us, whether as carbohydrates such as starch, or as lipids or fats, such as olive oil, and so on. Most of this type of phytochemical is also essential to the life of the plant and is usually referred to by plant scientists as a primary metabolite.

As such, these chemicals are produced principally in the green parts of the plant by photosynthesis. This essential set of chemical reactions converts carbon dioxide, water and sunlight into organic compounds. Many thousands of organic chemicals are produced by even the simplest of plants. Some of these organic compounds can have very powerful pharmacological effects when taken by mammals including humans. Because of this, many plants containing these active phytochemicals have a long history of use as medicines, initially in folklore, then in formalised systems of medicine.

Scientists spend a lot of time, money and use expensive sophisticated scientific equipment trying to unlock the phytochemical secrets of plants. Sometimes their quest is based on the arrogant belief that they can improve on the natural product. Sometimes they are simply curious and welcome the challenge of unravelling the chemical complexities produced by humble plants. Othertimes scientists would like to work with nature to bring effective reliable medicines within the reach of patients. In order to do so they need to know which chemicals are important and which are not. Armed with this knowledge they can choose the best plants, the best growing conditions, the best storage and handling conditions which will ensure that if one buys a valerian product this week one can be assured that it is of equal quality to the product bought a year ago and that it will be equally good when bought a year from now.

Given the widespread popularity of Valerian, it is not surprising that it has attracted a lot of attention from medicinal plant researchers. On the basis of what we know about the phytochemistry of Valerian or, more accurately, what we don't know, it might be appropriate to call this plant the Scarlet Pimpernel. This is because of the elusiveness of its active principles. Despite many hundreds of studies, it is not yet possible to definitively attribute the tranquillising, sedative effects to any particular group of phytochemicals produced by the Valerian plant. We can say that the effects are due to a mixture of chemicals some known and some as yet unknown.

Attention has been concentrated on two major groups of organic chemicals. The first is the volatile oil responsible for the unpleasant smell of Valerian. Like other more pleasant smelling volatile oils (so-called because they vapourise at room temperature as distinct from the non-volatile fatty oils such as sunflower oil which are known as fixed oils), Valerian oil is a very complex mixture of 12 monoterpenes and 17 sesquiterpenes. Monoterpenes have ten carbon atoms while sesquiterpenes have fifteen. In Valerian it is the *sesquiterpenes* which are important and which will appear again in our story. Names to watch out for include Valerenic acid, Valerenal and Valeranone. There are lots of

Valeriana species but only the "official" drug, Valerian, appears to contain Valerenic acids.

The second major group of compounds in Valerian are known as *valepotriates*. I know, I know, it is a mouthful but, as I tell my students, I don't think up the names! These chemicals, chief among them valtrate, are unstable, water insoluble compounds known in jargon terms as iridoids. This name is derived from the fact that the first iridoids were actually isolated from the venom of an ant which glories in the Latin name, Iridomyrmex. Here endeth (for the time being) what my children refer to as the 'actual factual' on the chemistry of Valerian.

Laboratory Tests

The development of a new drug usually tends to follow a set path from its discovery until it reaches the pharmacy. In testing its activity it is usual to have a series of what are called *in vitro* or test tube tests followed by *in vivo* studies in various laboratory animals leading ultimately to clinical trials in healthy volunteers and then in patients. In describing the evidence for the value of Valerian, that is normally the sequence I would have set out to follow. In this case however the *in vitro* testing of Valerian is a much more modern development and so I have chosen to describe events on a more or less chronological basis.

Testing Valerian as a Sedative

The testing of any drug as a sedative generally relies on observing changes in behaviour in animals treated with it. One example of such a test is to measure spontaneous movement in mice perhaps by means of an electronic counter. A sedative drug would reduce spontaneous movement in such a test. Another widely used test involves a comparison of the length an animal sleeps after being dosed with both a barbiturate and the test material compared to the sleeping time with barbiturate alone. Effective sedatives would prolong the barbiturate-induced sleeping time. Yet another test method measures impairment of co-ordination or motor function. The so-called 'Rotarod' test is a version of this, consisting of a rod which rotates at a speed such that control or undrugged animals can stay on it for at least 1 minute. Any herb or synthetic drug which affects motor function would cause the test animals to fall off the rod before the one minute was reached.

Research work on Valerian carried out during the early years of this century showed that tinctures did have sedative effects and this has been repeatedly confirmed since then. Initially it was thought that the foul-smelling oil was responsible, possibly in the time-honoured belief that if it tastes or smells vile it must be good for you. Studies during the 1950's and 1960's suggested that the oil could only account for about one third of the activity but consistently all of the researchers could demonstrate effects by measuring reductions in spontaneous movement and prolongation of sleeping time for various extracts and fractions.

The researchers kept investigating and eventually they struck gold in the form of the valepotriates (or so they thought!)

Valepotriates

When these chemically complex compounds were identified in Valerian in 1966 it was soon realised that they were highly significant in terms of the effects of Valerian and a standardised mixture was widely prescribed in what was then West Germany. Both animal tests and clinical trials showed the value of these compounds. For example, when given to cats it decreased their restlessness and anxiety. A major advantage of the valepotriates became apparent when researchers found that the toxicity of alcohol was not increased when mixed with them, whereas this was a significant risk when a benzodiazepine such as diazepam was mixed with alcohol.

The valepotriates however came under a cloud when experiments with cells grown artifically in test tubes showed that they could be damaged by valepotriates. This triggered off a temporary scare about Valerian, which has been shown to be totally unjustified on the basis that *in vivo* studies showed no significant damaging effect even at ludicrously high levels (1.3g/kilo of body weight) given orally. In addition, because these compounds are water insoluble and highly unstable, they are most unlikely to be detectable in finished preparations. Indeed, because of this latter fact, a number of medicinal plant researchers (myself included) were highly critical of the fact that most commercial Valerian products did not contain any valepotriates. In what became a curious reversal, a scientific test for the identity of Valerian based on the presence of valepotriates rapidly became a reassuring test for the absence of the same compounds!

The fact that the activity of Valerian declines with a corresponding decline in valepotriate content triggered off a number of studies. Some showed that decomposition products of the valepotriates were active, while others confirmed that some of the sesquiterpenes from the volatile oil were active.

Valeranone

A sesquiterpene present in Valerian but originally found in a plant called Nardostachys (the source of the 'Nard" of the Bible) was found to increase barbiturate induced sleeping time in mice. It was also found to be antispasmodic.

Valerenic Acid

Both valerenic acid and valerenal from the oil of Valerian showed significant effects on mice including a reduction in activity and decreased rotarod performance. In a follow-up study the effect of valerenic acid on the rotarod performance, on spontaneous motor activity and on sleeping time were further studied. Doses of about 60mg of valerenic acid reduced activity and prolonged the sleeping time. Higher doses adversely affected rotarod performance in a way that resembled a barbiturate. There is no doubt that valerenic acid is widely believed to be a most important constituent of the volatile oil of Valerian.

A difficulty arose however in trying to reconcile the activity of Valerian extracts which contained quite small amounts of these sesquiterpenes. This difficulty was highlighted when some very sophisticated experiments performed in 1986 and 1988 showed that solvent extracts of Valerian Root could depress the central nervous system. However tests using the same technique, involving the radioactive scanning of brain cells for glucose uptake, gave negative results, not only with the essential oil and its key components, but also with the valepotriates. The difficulty facing scientists working on Valerian is how to reconcile the conflicting results of the studies which show that extracts are effective in animals (and as will be seen in a later section) in humans but that studies of the key chemicals from the plant cannot account for the activity. One probable explanation which occurs to me is that there are other as yet unidentified compounds occurring in Valerian which are active. This seems probable when the effectiveness of aqueous extracts known to be devoid of valepotriates is taken into account. An additional piece of the jigsaw comes from a 1993 study in which a commercially available dried aqueous extract of Valerian was tested in mice using motility and sleeping time measurements. In each case there was a dose-related sedative effect which, while weaker than that obtained with diazepam, was still quite marked. This indicates that aqueous extraction of the roots does not damage or destroy the active principles in any way.

The final pieces of the jigsaw look as if they will be identified as a result of highly sophisticated tests using receptors found in brain cells. It seems ironic that what our ancestors have known for centuries should have to await scientific affirmation using the highest of high technology drug testing methods.

Valerian and Brain Receptors

The human brain is highly complex, intricate and elegantly assembled. We are still learning about how it controls all our activities, thoughts and moods. We know that much of its activity takes place at lightning speeds thanks to electrical impulses and various chemical transmitters which help carry signals within brain cells and from the brain to distant parts of the body.

In the case of Valerian, a key chemical is an amino-acid known as GABA. It is known that sedation in the central nervous system is strongly influenced by GABA which binds to specific receptors in brain cells, in much the same way as a key fits into a lock. GABA functions are known to be disrupted when people suffer from anxiety or depression and scientists are trying to design drugs which will bind to GABA receptors as a way of treating different neurological and psychiatric conditions.

In the last few years a number of research groups have been able to identify these GABA receptors and to isolate them for use in very sophisticated tests in the laboratory. Researchers in Italy and in Portugal have harnessed these high-tech methods to the study of Valerian. One group studied not only GABA receptors but also specific brain receptors for the well-known tranquilliser drugs, the benzodiazepines. They found that extracts of Valerian Root prepared with either water or mixtures of water and alcohol were able to bind to the GABA receptor. However the binding was not due to the sesquiterpenes or to the valepotriates, neither of which showed any affinity for the receptors.

Similar results were found at a laboratory in Portugal in experiments which indicated that aqueous extracts influenced the transport of GABA in key parts of nerve cells in a way that is consistent with the sedative properties. Because they found that Valerenic acid did not have any effect on GABA and because other researchers found little affinity for benzodiazepine receptors in the brain, the Portuguese group have begun to look for reasons why the total extracts bind to these key receptors but some compounds from the plant do not. They found that water extracts of the roots contain relatively high concentrations of amino-acids. Amino-acids are nitrogen containing chemicals which form the building blocks of proteins. In terms of brain chemistry GABA is a vital amino acid. The finding of good levels of GABA in those Valerian extracts is seen as having some significance. Even though the plant GABA cannot cross what is called the blood-brain barrier and thus cause sedation, it might be responsible for the relaxant properties of Valerian. The sedative effects could be explained by the presence in Valerian of another amino-acid called glutamine, because it can cross the blood-brain barrier and be taken up by nerve cells. Nerve cells can then convert glutamine into GABA and the increased levels would thus cause sedation.

Human Studies

The discovery of the valepotriates in the mid-60's led to a large number of clinical studies on either iridoid mixtures or purified compounds. These, as many subsequently realised, were of little relevance in the context of preparations containing powdered Valerian or made from aqueous extracts of the root, many of which contained little or no valepotriates. Indeed on a personal note, I was one of those who was highly critical of the quality of commercial Valerian preparations then available because none of them contained any valtrate etc. I am happy to admit that I got it wrong and what seemed to be a problem, actually turned out to be a probable advantage, given the (admittedly slight) query over the safety of the valepotriates.

Most of the recent clinical studies have used Valerian in which valepotriates were not a significant feature. A study by an Italian team led by Delsignore, published in 1980, looked at patients with mild anxiety and emotional tension. Half of the patients received a dummy placebo while the other twenty were given two Valerian tablets (50mg) three times a day. After three weeks it was obvious that Valerian had a positive effect and, given its absence of side effects, was deemed safe and effective in the treatment of emotional tension.

In 1981, Moser showed the value of a product containing both Valerian and hops (see Chapter 3) as a medicine to reduce stress in traffic. Significant improvement in both levels of stress and in reaction times was recorded. The importance of this study lies in the fact that it shows an important advantage of Valerian, namely that it did not appear to interfere with driving ability. The same cannot be said of the Benzodiazepine type drugs! However, given the attitude adopted by the German Health Authorities requiring warning labels, it is probably wiser to take refuge in the oft-repeated phrase beloved of drug scientists and say that "more studies are needed".

The Swiss Study

In my opinion the most important human studies of Valerian are those performed by Leathwood and Chauffard using an aqueous extract which they showed to be virtually free of valepotriates. This extract was studied in volunteers who filled in questionnaires and in volunteers who spent their nights in a sleep laboratory.

In all, 166 volunteers took part in the experiment. They were all given nine sets of capsules, three containing placebo, three containing the Valerian extract and three containing a mix of Valerian and Hops. They were also supplied with 9 questionnaires covering what is termed sleep latency (i.e. time taken to fall asleep), sleep quality, night awakening, dream recall and sleepiness the next morning. Each person was asked to take one set of capsules (coded so that they had no idea what they were taking) 1 hour before bedtime on non-consecutive nights and to fill in the questionnaire the next morning.

When the results of the questionnaires were analysed, Valerian was found to have produced a statistically significant increase in reports of reduced sleep latency (fig. 1).

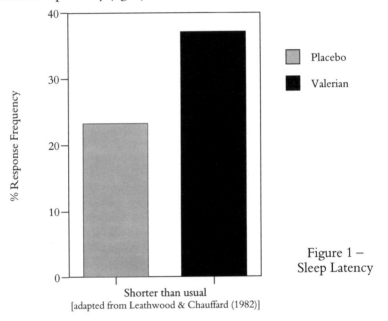

Figure 1 –
Sleep Latency

[adapted from Leathwood & Chauffard (1982)]

In other words the test subjects took less time to fall asleep. A more detailed analysis of the results indicated that sleep latency was most affected in older people, of whom 49% reported a beneficial effect.

As shown in fig. 2 (opposite), Valerian significantly improved the quality of sleep as reported by the human guinea pigs. Moreover a detailed analysis of the results showed that good sleepers gained little benefit but most importantly, poor or irregular sleepers had vastly improved sleep quality (fig. 3).

The most notable results in terms of better quality of sleep after taking

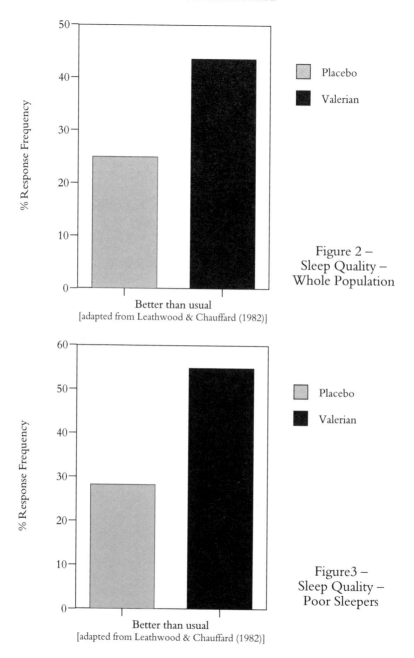

Figure 2 –
Sleep Quality –
Whole Population

[adapted from Leathwood & Chauffard (1982)]

Figure3 –
Sleep Quality –
Poor Sleepers

[adapted from Leathwood & Chauffard (1982)]

the Valerian capsules were from younger poor sleepers. Nearly two-thirds of older poor sleepers reported sleeping better than usual but a very high percentage (43%) of this group also reported good sleep quality after taking the placebo. Cigarette smokers accounted for one-third of the volunteers and, among those smokers, 52% reported better sleep quality after Valerian compared to 22% after placebo. Another positive result was that poor sleepers reported fewer night awakenings than usual after Valerian. In addition there was no increase in the frequency of reports of subjects being "more sleepy than usual" the following morning. The reason this question was included was to check if Valerian caused a "hangover" effect in the same way as benzodiazepines.

Summarising their results, Leathwood and Chauffard wrote that Valerian was active early in the night, that it improved sleep quality and produced no hangover after-effects the next day.

In a follow-up study the same researchers tested the same extract in 8 volunteers who suffered from mild insomnia. In order to provide more objective data, these volunteers were fitted with activity meters which are a standard way of estimating sleep latency and stability and sleeping time without interference with normal life. None of the volunteers reported any side effects during the 12 nights of the study. Again Valerian was compared with placebo. During the nights when the volunteers were using placebo capsules they took an average of 16 minutes to fall asleep. But Valerian yet again produced a significant decrease in the time taken to fall asleep from 16 down to 9 minutes. Doubling the dose had no further effect. The results showed that while Valerian produced more stable sleep than placebo during the first part of the night, it had no significant effect on total sleep time. Doubling the dose of Valerian extract up to 900mg increased reports of volunteers feeling more sleepy, suggesting that, with a high enough dose, a hangover effect is possible.

In their conclusions the authors point to a favourable comparison of the effects of Valerian on sleep latency compared to those of many benzodiazepines. Many of the benzodiazepines such as nitrazepam did shorten sleep latency and increase quality but at the expense of morning sleepiness. Leathwood and Chauffard, in their article in the prestigious scientific journal of medicinal plant research, Planta Medica (1985), go on to say "the changes we observe with Valerian suggest that it is at least as effective as small doses of barbiturates and benzodiazepines". To which I would add – and an awful lot safer!

Slightly contrary results were reported by other researchers in 1984. They found that after dosing 8 poor sleepers with a Valerian extract there was no effect on sleep latency but that there was an increase in slow-wave sleep. The following year another group studied the effects of an extract similar to that used by the Swiss team, on two groups of healthy young people at home. Those tested reported significant reductions in sleep latency and time awaking after they had fallen asleep. Laboratory studies which measured motor activity, sleep recordings and electrical activity in the brain (EEG) showed a similar trend.

The most recent clinical study to have appeared in the medico-scientific literature used a Valerian preparation standardised on its content of sesquiterpenes. Those enrolled in the test were volunteers with self-reported difficulties in sleeping. As is usual in these trials, neither the human subjects or the medical staff examining them knew whether they were receiving genuine Valerian or an inert dummy product resembling the Valerian. Nearly 90% of those given Valerian reported that their sleep had improved while 44% reported perfect sleep.

So, a story which began two millenia ago is still unfolding. There is a rich irony in the fact that modern science is only now beginning to confirm what generations of patients, herbalists and doctors have always known – if you need a good safe effective reliable sedative, Valerian not only fits the bill, it tops it.

2 | Also starring (from South America) the Passion Flower

Go on, be honest, what word pictures are conjured up by the expressions 'passion flower' and 'passion fruit'? I strongly suspect that sedation and tranquillising effects are not what most people associate with these terms!

The name 'passion flower' has always seemed to me to be totally misplaced, given that the leaves of Passiflora are actually used as a sedative rather than as an aphrodisiac. The name in fact comes from the supposed resemblance between the parts of the flower of Passiflora and the instruments used in the Passion or Crucifixion of Christ. In this symbolic association the three styles (part of the female section of the flower) represent the three nails, the ovary looks like a hammer, the corona looks like a crown of thorns and so on.

Originally Passiflora grew in South America but it is now cultivated as an ornamental in Europe and also for its exotic fragrant fruit in many countries. This passion fruit is produced from a number of varieties of *Passiflora edulis*, whereas the medicinally used plant is *Passiflora incarnata*, although other related species are used for instance in South America, e.g. *Passiflora coerulea*. In Europe this latter plant is of more interest to horticulturists than to herbalists.

The medicinal use of Passiflora is relatively recent, dating back to about 1867 in the USA. These plants came to Europe via the Spanish but were used first in homoeopathy especially in the treatment of sleep disturbances in patients suffering from neurasthenia, hysteria and nervous disorders. In the 1920's the French doctor Leclerc described the use of Passiflora and its extracts in the treatment of menopausal symptoms and as a medicine against insomnia.

A 1986 survey of herbal sedatives in the United Kingdom showed that Passiflora was the most popular herbal sedative based on its presence in the largest number of proprietary herbal medicines. Because of its popularity as a sedative, many scientists have tried to unlock the mystery of its effects. Much is known about the chemicals produced in the leaves. But there has always been an element of controversy surrounding Passiflora, not only in respect of its medicinal effects but also in respect of the chemicals it contains and their relationship to its sedative effects and in earlier years, its safety.

Nowadays, as a result of experiments using very sophisticated methods of phytochemical analysis there is general consensus that the major significant chemicals in Passion flower leaves are called flavonoids. Flavonoids are more famous perhaps as plant pigments but are also attracting more and more attention because of their strong antioxidant effects. Suffice it to say that Passiflora leaves contain up to 2.5 percent of a complex mixture of flavonoids with much much smaller amounts of chemicals such as maltol and cyanide-producing glycosides (0.01%). The low level of the latter is of course reassuring as is the recent finding that certain powerful compounds called Harman-alkaloids could not be detected in commercial plant material. Some years ago it had been suggested that these alkaloids were the active compounds, but on further study it was realised that this type of alkaloid was actually a stimulant and in high doses might even be hallucinogenic. It seems likely therefore that Polish reports in 1960 that both the alkaloid fraction and a flavonoid fraction had sedative actions were wrong.

Since then a veritable galaxy of international studies has been carried out on Passiflora, all supporting its use as a sedative but none conclusively, pinpointing the "active principle". In 1974 a Japanese team investigated Passiflora because of the adverse reactions of synthetic tranquillisers. They found that a fraction produced from the dry extract of the plant caused a slowing down of activity in mice as well as decreasing the uptake of oxygen by rat brain cells. This, they say, suggested that the extract contained sedative components. They then went on to isolate maltol from the Passiflora extract. Maltol has all the properties of a sedating compound with effects on the central nervous system; it decreased motor activity in mice at relatively low doses, it prolonged sleeping time in mice dosed with a barbiturate and also had anticonvulsant activity. The fly in the ointment, however, was the really small amount of maltol they found in the Passiflora. A concentration of only 0.05% meant that "it seems difficult to explain that the sedative effects of PIE [Passiflora incarnata Extract – authors note] are only due to Maltol."

1984 saw a Brazilian group investigating the related species *Passiflora alata* which was widely used in popular medicine as a sedative and tranquilliser and which was offically listed in the Brazilian Pharmacopoeia. They confirmed that extracts of the plant reduced motor activity and prolonged sleeping time in mice treated with barbiturates, as would be expected for a sedative material.

In 1988 two pharmaceutical scientists from the University of Bologna in Italy decided to investigate the effects of Passiflora extracts on the nervous system because of the fact that the active principles had still not been recognised. They subsequently reported that Passiflora has a complex action on the central nervous system. Yet again they obtained evidence for a sedative action which they said was due to at least two different chemical products. One of the active products was present in a very water soluble fraction which contained the majority of the flavonoid derivatives. Earlier workers had suggested these as likely candidates for the role of "active principles" but Speroni and Minghetti were quite definite in stating "but these compounds can be ruled out as responsible for the activity" because they were inactive when tested as pure compounds.

Another Italian study published in 1990 measured a 57% reduction in spontaneous activity in rats after treatment with a Passiflora tincture while a number of German and Swiss studies published in 1993 and 1994 add weight to the sizeable body of pharmacological evidence that Passiflora is an effective sedative and anti-anxiety agent.

The Benzodiazepine Connection

It is generally accepted that the ever-increasing popularity of herbal sedatives and tranquillisers is due to the public awareness of the risks of the synthetic benzodiazepines which are the cornerstone of conventional medical responses to stress, insomnia and anxiety. It is ironic therefore that some of the most sophisticated research support for the activity of Passiflora has come from investigations into benzodiazepines. These benzodiazepines, or BZD's in shorthand jargon, were discovered by chance in 1957 and for a long time were considered to be non-natural products until 1986 when they were discovered in rat, bovine and human brains. It was then discovered that these BZD's were present in plasma, milk, wheat grains and several plants. Eventually receptors capable of binding benzodiazepine drugs were found to exist in the human brain. Receptors are a key concept in modern drug research because drugs, whether produced in a test tube or in a bacterium or in a plant leaf, are believed to work by fitting into receptor sites in a manner similar to the way a key fits into a lock. Once bound to the receptor site, which could be in any cell in any part of the body, the drug could either cause an effect or it could block an existing natural effect. Large numbers of receptors have now been identified and in many cases isolated. In many respects they have dramatically changed our view of how the body works. For example, the identification of the morphine receptors in the body led to the identification of the body's own painkillers, the enkephalins and endorphins. More recently the African arrow poison, ouabain, has been identified as the human body's own digitalis molecule which binds to digitalis receptors in the heart. But to return to the benzodiazepines or BZD's, receptors which specifically bind these molecules exist in the brain and these can be isolated and used to test the ability of chemicals and plant extracts to bind to their sites. This binding can be measured very accurately, minutely using very small sub microscopic amounts of drug labelled radioactively.

An Argentinian group decided to test plants used in South America in folk medicine as tranquillisers or mild sedatives. They included a Passiflora species (*P. coerulea*) in their test. All of the plants examined contained substances which bound to BZD-receptors but the Passiflora and Tilia (lime flower) were particularly noteworthy. Subsequent experiments with the Passiflora sample showed that several active compounds were detected rather than any single potential 'magic bullet'. However in time-honoured fashion one compound called chrysin was isolated and identified as having significant capacity to bind to benzodiazepine receptors. Unusually it had no nitrogen, being a flavonoid compound. Chrysin was then tested in mice and found to have effects consistent with an anti-anxiety effect similar to that produced by diazepam (Valium®). The Argentinian scientists went on to state that the data from extensive tests suggested that chrysin was an anxiolytic but that it did not induce sedation or muscle relaxation.

The situation is therefore not at all clear cut. Firstly chrysin has not been detected in *Passiflora incarnata*, which is the plant used in Europe, although it contains other flavonoids which could also bind to the brain receptors. Secondly the amounts of the benzodiazepine-like molecules found in these herbal sedatives are probably lower than the levels needed to exert a drug effect. However it has recently been suggested that the long term intake of trace amounts of BZD's could cause an increase in the levels of BZD's in brain cells. Thus, it has beeen suggested, it is entirely feasible that chronic, i.e. long term, intake of the plant compounds could similarly influence brain function.

It is therefore still too soon to write a conclusion to the Passiflora story. It becomes more and more complex as we learn more about the plant, its chemistry and its biological effects and as we learn more about the intricacies of the human brain and nervous system. The scientific research to date leaves little doubt about the value of Passiflora, even though evidence from that Holy Grail of medico-scientific research, the clinical trial in humans, is lacking.

The Official View

Whatever about the detailed scientific experiments, the Health authorities in at least three European countries recognise Passiflora as a sedative. In Germany the influential Kommission E of the German Health Office drew up a monograph on Passiflora herb in 1985 and amended it in 1990. This official monograph states that Passiflora is used for nervous restlessness on the basis that in experimental research on animals a slowing down of mobility has been repeatedly observed.

The French Government published extensive guidelines on the marketing of plant medicines (phytomedicines) in 1990 in which two key lists appeared; one a list of accepted plant drugs and the other a list of accepted indications or medical conditions which could be treated by the listed plants. In the case of Passiflora it is listed as being traditionally used to reduce excitability in adults and children, particularly in cases of disorders of sleep.

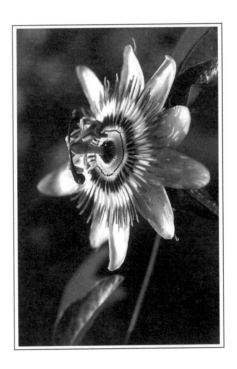

3 | In which we meet a bitter member of the supporting cast

Mention *Humulus lupulus* to most beer drinkers and almost certainly their response will vary from polite incomprehension through to impolite expletives. Mention Hops, on the other hand, and visions of Kent and of the Darling Buds of May are evoked, the taste buds primed for another pint of best bitter and all is understood, because *Humulus lupulus* is the Latin botanical name for those hops without which beer wouldn't taste like beer.

Hops were first cultivated by the Romans and surprisingly only spread to England in the 16th century. The Hop plant is a unisex plant with some plants producing male flowers and some producing female flowers. The female flowers are small green fircone shaped catkins known as strobiles. The papery scales cover small yellow glands which contain the hop bitters so essential to the brewer's art as they impart flavour, aroma and improve the keeping properties of the beer. These strobiles are picked in late summer and gently dried before being used in brewing.

Folklore has it that the medicinal sedative properties of hops was first noticed among hop pickers. Legend indicates that hop pickers tired easily, as a result, it was said, of the transfer of hop resin from their hands to their mouths. Initially hop pillows were used for sleeplessness and nervous ailments, subsequently extracts, tinctures, even the sifted glands known as lupulin, were and still are used as medicines, under such aliases as 'Humulus', 'Lupulus', 'Lupuli strobili' etc.

A Chemical Cocktail

Because of the economic importance of hops, there has been enormous scientific interest in its chemical composition and attempts have been made to improve the amounts of flavour components through plant breeding, biotechnology and good agricultural practice. Like most plants Humulus is an incredibly inventive chemical factory producing many different types of organic compounds (in what still seems to me a miraculous way) from carbon dioxide, water and sunlight.

From a beer drinker's perspective (and I include myself in that description), the most important hop chemicals are the 15-25% resinous bitter principles made up mainly of a mixture of α-acids such as humulone and β-acids such as lupulone. The chemical cocktail (alcohol-free at this stage!) also contains a volatile oil, flavonoids and phenolic compounds.

The bitter principles are strongly antibacterial but also extremely unstable in air and light. One scientist has estimated that hops could lose up to 85% of its activity after only nine months storage. This is unfortunate for professional and amateur brewers alike but, according to one theory, may be vital to attempts to explain the medicinal use of the plant.

Many attempts have been made to identify the chemicals in hops which might cause sedative effects. Many of the results of early studies are complicated by the fact that animals such as frogs and golden carp were used – how the scientists performing these tests hoped to extrapolate their results to human beings is beyond me! In addition, many more orthodox tests involved using hops in combination with other plants, especially Valerian. Again it is nigh impossible to establish if the positive results owe anything to the hops or if they are only due to the Valerian. The best that can be said about the early work is that it showed that the bitter acids were not the sedative agents.

In 1967 a volatile compound, methylbutenol, was isolated and is believed to be one of the key compounds in terms of sedative properties. Only traces of this compound were detected in fresh hops but amounts increased continuously after drying to reach a peak of about 0.15% after two years at ordinary temperatures. There is however reason to believe that methylbutenol may also be formed *in vivo* (i.e. inside the cells of the body) from the bitter α-acids such as humulone which are present in much larger amounts in the hops.

This methylbutenol was then tested for its soporific (sleep-inducing) effects and preliminary results showed that in mice it produced sleep for about 8 hours. It was further studied in rats in whom it caused a 50% reduction in motility within two minutes. This effect, interpreted as a central nervous depressant effect, reached a maximum after two hours.

The effectiveness of the methylbutenol was compared with that of a known sedative drug of synthetic origin called methylpentynol. This latter drug is chemically very similar to the hop chemical and has been marketed under the trade names Insomnol® and Oblivon® (where do they get the names from?). It was found that both substances were effective sedatives within the same dose range.

That, you might think, finished the story, but you would be wrong. It has been calculated that a single effective dose of methylbutenol would require all of 150 grammes of hops. On this basis, the methylbutenol naturally present in the hops could only partially explain the value of hops. Metabolism of the bitters might add a little more but probably could not account for all of the activity. The situation has still not been clarified conclusively. Some believe that the hops aroma may help the relaxation process, possibly through a direct action on the olfactory centres (responsible for smell perception) and thus on the central nervous system. Given the value of aromatherapy in relaxation this is certainly an attractive theory. Another explanation could lie hidden in those benzodiazepine receptors which were described in the previous chapter.

According to the British Herbal Compendium monograph, hops contain a minimum of 0.5% of flavonoids including some which have been shown to bind to benzodiazepine receptors in the brain. It is not inconceivable that scientists have let their taste buds blind them to the possibility that components other than the resins and bitters might be responsible for the effects traditionally ascribed to hops.

In France, Germany and Belgium there is official acceptance by the relevant health authorities that hops have value as a sleeping herb. In the French "Avis aux fabricants" or government notice to manufacturers of herbal medicines, hops can be marketed provided it is labelled as being "traditionally used to reduce excitability in adults and children, particularly in cases of disorders of sleep". In Germany the Komission E which was given the task of reviewing the scientific evidence on hundreds of medicinal plants, has published a monograph on hops which accepts that hops could be used in "disturbed states such as restlessness and anxiety and disorders of sleep". It specifically notes that combinations with other sedative drugs might be advantageous and, as we shall see in the next chapter, there is no shortage of candidates for inclusion in such combinations.

4 | The supporting cast

Over the years many plants have gained a reputation as being useful sedatives and tranquillising medicines. Some of these are briefly described in this chapter.

Motherwort

As the English name suggests, Motherwort has long had a reputation as a herb for female illnesses and as the latin name, Cardiaca, indicates, it was recommended as a herb which gladdened and strengthened the heart. However it also is reputed as a nervine and sedative herb. Motherwort is not a plant which has been extensively studied in recent years. A related species, Siberian Motherwort, was investigated in 1986 and showed some evidence of sedative activity in laboratory tests. These tests also showed that it was of low toxicity.

It has been reported that a chemical called apigenin which is a key ingredient in German Chamomile, is also present in Motherwort and more recently (1995) it has been shown that this apigenin has the ability to bind to benzodiazepine receptors. While this in no way 'proves' that Motherwort is a sedative plant, it does strengthen the case for it

Chamomile

As just mentioned, apigenin is a key component of the water soluble fraction of German Chamomile (Matricaria), one of the best loved of herbs. While its main claim to fame is its use in stomach ailments and as an antiinflammatory healing agent in skin complaints, Chamomile tea also has a reputation as a mild relaxing aid to sleep. Studies in the 1980's showed that Chamomile flowers did slow down the nervous system. Exactly how this effect might occur has become clearer as a result of work carried out in Argentina and reported in a key scientific journal devoted to research into medicinal plants. These workers reported that they had detected several fractions from a water extract of the plant (i.e. Chamomile tea) which had the ability to bind to benzodiazepine receptors. Subsequent experiments identified apigenin as having anti-anxiety effects and a slight sedative effect. It is perhaps ironic that this scientific support for the traditional folk use of this plant has had to await the development of some of the scientifically most advanced methods of testing. It appears increasingly that 'scientific proof' for many phytomedicines only comes when scientific methods can actually test the herbs properly.

Lemon Balm

This is one of my favourite herbs. Indeed if the concept of a "desert island herb garden" did not seem such a contradiction, Melissa or Balm mint, as this plant is also called, would be one of my prime candidates ; (the others would include Chamomile, Echinacea, Ginseng, Garlic, Valerian, Basil – to which I confess an addiction – Sage and Ginger), partly because of its beautiful smell, partly because of the refreshing calming tea and partly because of its beneficial healing effects on cold sores. Lemon balm is also widely used to treat tenseness, restlessness and general irritability. A number of laboratory studies have shown that it has a sedative effect.

There has always been a strong tradition of using mixtures of these sleeping herbs. Scientific support for such mixtures can sometimes be lacking. One study published in mid 1995 examined the value of a phytosedative mixture containing extracts from Valerian, Hops and Lemon Balm. The authors tested the preparation on 225 patients who reported difficulty in falling asleep and remaining asleep during the night. After two weeks there was a significant improvement on the severity of the symptoms. 89% of patients reported that difficulty in falling asleep had improved and difficulty in sleeping through the night had improved in 80% of patients.

Other Sedative Herbs

A number of other herbs appear in the herbal literature as being useful in helping to obtain a good night's rest. Dr. Rudolf Weiss, who was probably the most influential medical doctor specialising in Phytotherapy over the past 20 years, mentions the use of oats as a drink in milk. He notes that the virtues of oats should be taken seriously and should be further studied. Weiss also mentions Californian Poppy.

Californian Poppy

The yellow orange flower of *Eschscholtzia californica*, known as the Californian poppy, is the State flower of California. Although it is a member of the poppy family it does not produce morphine-type alkaloids. Instead it contains alkaloids similar to those found in *Sanguinaria* (Bloodroot). Traditionally used by the native American Indians as a painkiller and sedative, Escholtzia was introduced into Europe because of its ornamental flowers.

Nowadays this plant is prescribed in France as a sedative. A French research group tested an aqueous extract in mice after first determining that the extract had no toxic effects in the mice. They found that their experimental results validated the traditional sedative properties. They further discovered that the Californian Poppy appeared to have an anxiolytic (anti-anxiety) effect. While no standard clinical trials have yet been reported for this plant, a number of case reports from French medical doctors specialising in phytotherapy have been published. In one case a 32 year old married woman presented to her G.P. with insomnia of several months duration; after 3 weeks treatment with a tincture of the Californian poppy her sleep pattern had returned to normal. Similar results were recorded in the case of a 44 year-old male after one month. This particular G.P. also reported a 60% improvement in 150 patients suffering from insomnia.

Because this plant is known to contain alkaloids which by definition are pharmacologically active and which can be quite powerful in their effects on the body, the question of safety arises. Studies in France indicate that it was not possible to determine a lethal toxic dose of either the tincture or the plant due to a lack of toxicity. It would seem that for most people this is another relatively safe herb though I would caution pregnant women against its use on principle and, the alkaloids have not been fully tested and thus might not be totally safe during pregnancy.

Lime Tree Flowers

Lime or Linden flowers and leaves constitute another traditional folk tea with a reputation for its calming influence just before bedtime. There are many species of Tilia (the botanical designation for the Lime tree) used to prepare such teas. One Tilia species has recently been shown to contain components which bind to those benzodiazepine receptors which have been mentioned several times already. Detailed scientific "proof" in terms of classical double blind clinical trials will probably never become available although two French G.P.'s have extolled the virtues of Lime buds. In one detailed case study they reported on a 38 year old woman who came to their surgery very anxious, exhausted through lack of sleep and having lost over 8 kilos in six months, due to tension and anxiety. At that time she was using both barbiturates and Diazepam, a well-known benzodiazepine. After taking the prescribed Tilia for one month, the patient rapidly stopped taking the barbiturates because her sleep had normalised and she had been able to halve the dose of diazepam due to a reduction in anxiety. After a further month she had totally abandoned the use of the Diazepam and the sole cause of anxiety now was the 4 kg in weight she had regained!

Wild Lettuce

This particular plant flourished as a sedative and painkiller in conventional American medicine for over a century from 1799 in the form of Lettuce Opium or, to give it its latin name, Lactucarium. This consists of the dried milky juice or latex of several species of lettuce, particularly the wild lettuce *Lactuca virosa*. The initial use of this drug as a sedative by the ancient Egyptians was probably influenced by the similarity in appearance, smell and taste of lactucarium to Opium which is the dried milky latex from the botanically unrelated Opium Poppy. Thankfully Lettuce Opium does not contain any of the morphine type alkaloids found in Opium. Research work in the 1930's showed that the action of Lettuce Opium could be attributed to the presence of bitter substances in the latex. A 1986 study from Puerto Rico, where lettuce juice has been used in traditional folk medicine for a long time, reported that a chemical agent with depressant effects was isolated from the stem of the garden lettuce, *Lactuca sativa*. The difficulty with this study is that the tests were carried out on toads and one must query how relevant toad physiology is to humans! It would be interesting to see the results of tests using the super-sophisticated test-tube tests now in vogue, to see if this most ancient of plant drugs actually has the effects ascribed to it down through the ages. This could prove worthwhile since the British Herbal Compendium lists apigenin as a constituent of Wild Lettuce. As mentioned under Chamomile this apigenin has very interesting effects.

The French Government in the meantime allows both Lime flowers and Wild Lettuce to be used, provided they are labelled as being "traditionally used to reduce nervousness in adults, notably in cases of minor sleep disorders."

5 | A sense of proportion

"Our revels now are ended. These our actors . . . are such stuff as dreams are made on, and our little life is rounded with a sleep" (with apologies to W. Shakespeare).

There are alternatives to the benzodiazepines. One alternative is to use one or more of the herbs described in the preceding chapters. Sometimes a change in lifestyle may be needed.

There is little doubt that nature provides us with a wide choice of sleeping herbs which may be of benefit to those seeking a restful night's sleep. However a sense of proportion is, as ever, vital. Just as the concept of the chemical "Magic bullet", which claims to cure all ills and solve all of life's problems, is an illusion, so too is the belief that "natural" herbs are miracle cures for every conceivable ailment known to mankind. The famous French herbalist, Maurice Messegue, probably hit the nail on the head when he wrote – "It is solely in the case of benign ailments, above all of chronic ailments, or in order to help in the treatment of serious illness that I recommend the use of herbs. See your doctor whenever it becomes necessary. To trust in Nature does not mean that you must deprive yourself of the discoveries of science."

6 | A reassurance about safety

All medicines, whether natural or synthetic, should be as safe as possible. However it is simply not possible to produce a 100 percent risk-free medication. By and large plant medicines are less toxic but it is important to bear in mind that the plant kingdom can produce some very nasty toxic chemicals such as strychnine, morphine, among others.

With regard to the plants mentioned in this book, their safety profiles are very high. Safety assessment by various European Governments clearly indicates that there are no known contra indications (i.e. situations where the herb should not be taken), side-effects or interactions with other drugs.

The scientific studies confirm these assessments. In one study of the toxicity of Valerian it was found that the essential oil was the least toxic of 27 commonly used essential oils including peppermint oil. Even very high levels of Valerian extract show very low levels of toxicity.

Valerian is not only exceptionally safe in terms of overdoses, it also has major advantages in that experiments show that it does not magnify the harmful effects of alcohol in the same way as conventional tranquillisers. In fact, one study of this aspect showed that Valerian actually antagonised the action of alcohol. Another major advantage lies in the fact that no evidence of any dependence syndrome developing to Valerian has ever been reported. This also applies to all the other herbs.

Some years ago concern was expressed that some combination products containing Valerian were implicated in a small number of cases of hepatitis. A detailed analysis of these cases did not provide any conclusive evidence linking Valerian in particular to adverse effects on the liver. The safety of Valerian in this respect was highlighted by a study reported in 1991 in which extremely high doses of Valerian extract (600mg for each kilogram of body weight) were tested. There was no difference between test and control animals in terms of either organ weights or haematological and biochemical parameters. In particular tests of liver function were identical between the two groups.

In the case of the other herbs many of them, e.g. lettuce and hops, are more widely used in the food and brewing industry and are explicitly approved for food use. The best way to illustrate the relative safety of all these plants is to use the comparison developed by an American authority which rates the safety of herbs by equating them to the safety of cups of coffee. It must be highly reassuring that hops, lettuce, motherwort, passiflora and valerian are all rated as being as safe as two cups of coffee per day!

7 | Further reading

In preparing this book I have tried to summarise a large amount of phytochemical, pharmacological and clinical data on sedative herbs in jargon-free (where possible) English. I have drawn on a large number of reviews and technical papers in doing so. Much of what is included comes from some key scientific publications and these are listed below.

Valerian

• The biological activity of Valerian and related plants. P.J. Houghton. *Journal of Ethnopharmacology* 22: 121-142 1988.
• Valerian – A literature review. C. Hobbs. *Herbalgram* No. 21: 20-34 1989.
• Valerian – Valeriana officinalis. S. Foster. American Botanical Council 1990.
• Valeriana officinalis: traditional use and recent evaluation of activity. P. Morazzoni and E. Bombardelli: *Fitoterapia* LXVI No. 2: 99-112 1995.
• Synaptosomal GABA Release as influenced by Valerian Root extract – involvement of the GABA carrier. *Arch. Int. Pharmacodyn* 327: 220-231. 1994.
• Aqueous extract of Valerian Root (Valeriana officinalis L) improves sleep quality in man. Leathwood P.D. et al. *Pharmacology Biochemistry and Behaviour* 17: 65-71 1982.
• Aqueous extract of Valerian reduces latency to fall asleep in man. Leathwood P D and Chauffard F. *Planta Medica* 1985: 144-148.

Passiflora

• Passiflora incarnata L – Passionsblume portrait einer arzneipflanze. B. Meier. *Zeit. für Phytotherapie* 16: 115-126 1995.
• British Herbal Compendium. P. Bradley (Editor). BHMA 1992.
• Neuropharmacological activity of extracts from Passiflora incarnata. E. Speroni and A. Minghetti. *Planta Medica* 54: 488-491 1988.

• Possible anxiolytic effects of Chrysin, a central benzodizepine receptor ligand isolated from Passiflora coerulea. Wolfman C et al. *Pharmacology Biochemistry and Behaviour* 47: 1-4 1994.

Hops

• Sedative and Hypnogenic effects of Hops. Stocker H R. *Schweizer Brauerei Rundschau*. 78: 80-89 1967.

• The sedative-hypnotic principles of Hops 3. Communication: Contents of 2-methyl-3-buten-2-ol in hops and hop preparations. R. Hänsel et al. *Planta Medica* 45: 224-228 1982.

• The sedative-hypnotic principles of Hops 4. Communication: Pharmacology of 2-methyl-3-buten-2-ol. R. Wohlfart et al. *Planta Medica* 48: 120-123 1983.

Other Sedative Herbs

• Behavioural effects of the American traditional plant Eschscholzia californica: sedative and anxiolytic properties. A. Rolland et al. *Planta Medica* 57: 212-216 1992.

• Neurotropic action of the hydroalcholic extract of *Melissa officinalis* in the Mouse. Soulimani R et al. *Planta Medica* 57: 105-109 1991.

• Apigenin: a component of Matricaria recutita flowers is a central benzodiazepine receptors – ligand with anxiolytic properties. H. Viola et al. *Planta Medica* 61: 213-216 1995.

• Isolation of Pharmacologically active benzodiazepine receptor ligands from Tilia tomentosa (Tiliaceae). H. Viola et al. *Journal of Ethnopharmacology* 44: 47-53 1994.

• Depressant Pharmacological effects of component isolated from lettuce *Lactuca sativa*. F. Gonzalex-Lima et al. *Int. J. Crude Drug Res.* 24: 154-166. 1986.

• Herbal Medicine. R F Weiss. A.B. Arcanum Gothenburg Sweden 1988. pages 280-291.

OTHER AMBERWOOD HEALTH TITLES INCLUDE:

Aromatherapy – A Guide for Home Use by Christine Westwood. All you need to know about essential oils and using them. £1.99.

Aromatherapy – For Stress Management by Christine Westwood. Covering the use of essential oils for everyday stress-related problems. £2.99.

Aromatherapy – For Healthy Legs and Feet by Christine Westwood. A comprehensive guide to the use of essential oils for the treatment of legs and feet, including illustrated massage instructions. £2.99.

Plant Medicine – A Guide for Home Use by Charlotte Mitchell MNIMH. A guide to home use giving an insight into the wonderful healing qualities of plants. £2.99.

Woman Medicine – Vitex Agnus Castus by Simon Mills MA, FNIMH. The wonderful story of the herb that has been used for centuries in the treatment of women's problems. £2.99.

Ancient Medicine – Ginkgo Biloba by Dr Desmond Corrigan BSc(Pharms), MA, Phd, FLS, FPSI. Improved memory, circulation and concentration are associated in this book with medicine from this fascinating tree. £2.99.

Indian Medicine – The Immune System by Desmond Corrigan BSc(Pharms), MA, Phd, FLS, FPSI. An intriguing account of the history and science of the plant called Echinacea and its power to influence the immune system. £2.99.

Herbal First Aid by Andrew Chevallier BA, MNIMH. A beautifully clear reference book of natural remedies and general first aid in the home. £2.99.

Natural Taste – Herbal Teas, A Guide for Home Use by Andrew Chevallier BA, MNIMH. This beautifully illustrated book contains a comprehensive compendium of Herbal Teas giving information on how to make it, its benefits, history and folklore. £2.99.

Signs & Symptoms of Vitamin Deficiency by Dr Leonard Mervyn BSc, PhD, C.Chem, FRCS. A home guide for self diagnosis which explains and assesses Vitamin Therapy for the prevention of a wide variety of diseases and illnesses. £2.99.

Causes & Prevention of Vitamin Deficiency by Dr Leonard Mervyn BSc, PhD, C.Chem, FRCS. A home guide to the Vitamin content of foods and the depletion caused by cooking, storage and processing. It includes advice for those whose needs are increased due to lifestyle, illness etc. £2.99.

Eyecare Eyewear – For Better Vision by Mark Rossi Bsc, MBCO. A complete guide to eyecare and eyewear including an assessment of the types of spectacles and contact lenses available and the latest corrective surgical procedures. £3.99.